Coronary Artery Disease (CAD) Recipe Cookbook

The Ultimate Life Changing Cookbook for Heart Disease and A Culinary Symphony for Coronary Wellness

Dr. Mary K. Clubb

This book is a work of non-fiction. All of the characters, incidents, and dialogue are drawn from the author's personal experiences, interviews, and research. Any resemblance to actual persons, living or dead, or events is entirely coincidental.

While the author has made every effort to provide accurate and up-to-date information, neither the author nor the publisher can be held responsible for any errors or omissions or for any consequences resulting from the use of this information.

Table Of Content

Introduction

A young lady called Emma lived in the vibrant metropolis of Heartsville, where life appeared to be going at an uncontrollable pace. She was enthusiastic, driven, and in constant motion. She had no idea that a diagnosis that would completely alter her life and cause her to undergo a spectacular metamorphosis was waiting for her in the hospital's hallways.

Emma was faced with the unexpected reality of Coronary Artery Disease (CAD) one day in the usual course of things. Her daily routine abruptly came to a grinding stop, and she realized she desperately needed to adopt a new outlook on life that put her heart health first.

A ray of hope appeared in the shape of a cookbook designed for those new to CAD and needing help understanding its intricacies. Emma leafed over its pages and found recipes and a guide to taking back control of her health. The cookbook became a traveling companion, helping her navigate the complex world of heart-healthy nutrition and giving her the confidence to make wise decisions.

There were difficulties along the way. Emma had periods of uncertainty and temptation but felt a fresh energy after mastering each dish. Once unfamiliar, the kitchen turned into her haven of recovery and self-discovery.

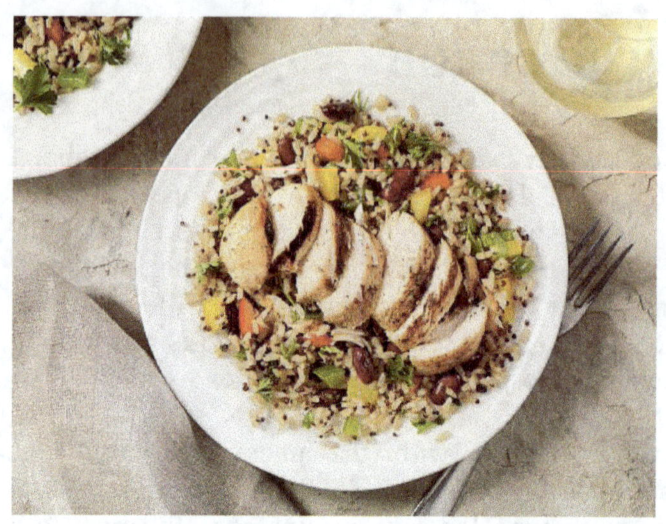

Emma learned about the resiliency of the human spirit and the sustaining power of food via her culinary explorations. She enjoyed cooking delectable dishes that nourished her heart as much as her taste senses. The smell of healthy cooking filled her kitchen, signifying the inward metamorphosis she was going through on a physical, mental, and spiritual level.

Emma's journey—from diagnosis to empowerment, uncertainty to renewed wellbeing—is chronicled in this book. Anyone dealing with the difficulties of CAD is invited to set off on their life-changing journey. These pages include more than simply recipes—they also tell a story of resiliency, hope, and the amazing potential of adopting a heart-healthy lifestyle.

This book serves as a beacon of hope for anyone looking to improve their heart health, showing them that achieving a healthy heart is feasible and can be a fulfilling, flavorful experience despite obstacles.

Chapter One
Understanding Coronary Artery Disease

1.1 Overview of Coronary Artery Disease (CAD)

Overview of Coronary Artery Disease (CAD): Navigating the Cardiovascular Health Labyrinth

Within the complex field of human health, Coronary Artery Disease (CAD) is a problem that affects millions of people globally and has the power to change the course of countless lives. Imagine the heart as a grand city, with its arteries representing the essential thoroughfares that sustain the life of the busy metropolis. Imagine now that these artery channels are blocked, preventing the heart from receiving the nutrition and oxygen it needs to survive.

Fundamentally, CAD is a disease marked by the constriction or occlusion of these vital arteries, often due to plaque buildup, a combination of fat, cholesterol, and other materials. The very core of life, the heart, is in danger as these once-clear passageways narrow.

However, CAD is more than just a medical diagnosis; it's a story that develops uniquely in each person. A warning sign that the heart, the conductor of life's symphony, needs treatment may begin as a faint murmur, mild discomfort during exercise, or appear as abrupt, severe pain.

This introduction acts as a compass, assisting you in navigating the routes to heart health and helping you comprehend the vocabulary and intricacies of the CAD labyrinth. We'll go into the science behind preventative tactics, examine the risk factors that throw doubt on these crucial arteries and stress the critical role diet plays in controlling and lessening the effects of CAD.

As we begin our investigation, remember that information is a means of gaining power and taking back control of your cardiovascular health. Come with me as we explore the heart's passageways, where learning about CAD is the foundation for creating a future replete with vigor, resiliency, and the steady beat of a healthy heart.

1.2 Risk Elements and Preventive Measures

Risk Factors and Proactive Approaches: Handling the Intersection of Heart Health

Knowing the risk factors for Coronary Artery Disease (CAD) becomes critical in the complex dance between our lifestyle choices and heart health. Consider these risk factors as roadside signposts that indicate possible detours toward cardiovascular difficulties. Let's explore the subtleties of these risk factors as we embark on our adventure and choose the best route for preventative measures.

1. Genetics and Age:

Risk Factor: As we age, we become more vulnerable to coronary artery disease (CAD). Aging is an essential part of life. Genetics also has a significant influence; a family history of heart disease might increase the risk.

Prevention Strategy: Being informed is essential even if we have no control over our age or genetic makeup. Frequent tests become necessary to decrease inherited risks via early intervention and lifestyle modifications.

2. Elevated Blood Pressure:

Risk factor: High blood pressure strains the arteries, increasing their vulnerability to deterioration and plaque buildup.

A heart-healthy diet, regular exercise, stress reduction, and, where required, medicines under medical supervision are all part of the prevention strategy.

3. Elevated Cholesterol:

Risk factor: High blood cholesterol impedes blood flow by causing plaque to accumulate in the arteries.

Prevention Strategy: Eating a diet high in omega-3 fatty acids and low in trans and saturated fats and frequent exercise helps keep cholesterol levels at their ideal range.

4. Smoking:

Risk factor: Smoking tobacco releases toxic compounds into the blood, hastening the onset of coronary artery disease (CAD).

Prevention Strategy: It's critical to stop smoking. A smoke-free path involves support networks, therapy, and lifestyle modifications that enable the body to heal and renew.

5. Diabetes:

Risk factor: Uncontrolled diabetes raises the chance of coronary artery disease (CAD) by causing blood vessel damage.

Preventive strategy: controlling blood sugar levels with a healthy diet, consistent exercise, and following prescription guidelines while under medical supervision.

6. Lack of Physical Activity:

Sedentary behavior damages the heart and makes other risk factors worse.

Prevention Strategy: Including regular exercise, even in small doses, improves heart health in general. Minor lifestyle adjustments like cycling or walking might have a significant influence.

7. Overweight:

Risk Factor: Being overweight puts undue strain on the heart and raises the risk of diabetes, high cholesterol, and high blood pressure.

Prevention Strategy: Maintaining a healthy weight requires a multimodal strategy that includes regular exercise, a balanced diet, and behavioral adjustments.

While these risk factors are potent foes, navigating the crossroads of heart health requires realizing that their effects may be lessened via education and preventative action. Making empowered decisions daily, working with your healthcare team, and traveling the path toward prevention is a team effort. The road to a heart-healthy existence becomes more apparent with knowledge, dedication, and persistence, and you are invited to walk boldly in the direction of a time when your heart beats robustly and in tune.

1.3 Nutrition's Significance in the Management of CAD

Nutrition's Role in Controlling Coronary Artery Disease (CAD): Increasing Heart Resilience

Nutrition is a critical player in the symphony of variables that affect our heart health; the conductor arranges the notes for a beautiful song of health. Recognizing the role nutrition plays in managing Coronary Artery Disease (CAD) is analogous to understanding the role that high-performance fuel plays in an engine. Let's examine the nuances of this link and how dietary decisions may play a significant role in the control and avoidance of CAD.

Heart-Healthy Fats:

Relevance: Not all fat is made equal. Avocados, fatty salmon, olive oil, and other foods high in mono- and polyunsaturated fats help lower cholesterol and promote cardiovascular health.

Management Strategy: Make these good fats the primary source of fat in your diet by substituting them for processed and fried meals that include trans and saturated fats. Use cooking techniques like baking, grilling, or steaming to preserve the nutritious value of your food.

The Fatty Acids Omega-3:

Significance: Rich in fish (salmon, mackerel, and flaxseeds), omega-3 fatty acids have anti-inflammatory qualities and promote heart health in general.

Management Strategy: Eat fatty fish at least twice a week. Walnuts, chia seeds, and flaxseeds are good non-fish sources. Supplements containing omega-3 may be advised under physician supervision.

Foods High in Fiber:

Dietary fiber, including whole grains, fruits, vegetables, and legumes, is crucial because it helps people maintain a healthy weight and decrease cholesterol.

Management Tip: Include a variety of foods high in fiber in your meals. At least five servings of fruits and vegetables should be consumed daily, and whole grains should be preferred over processed ones.

Trim Proteins:

Relevance: Lean protein sources, which don't include the extra saturated fats in certain meats, such as chicken, fish, beans, and lentils, provide vital amino acids.

Management Strategy:
- Choose lean meats.
- Include plant-based proteins in your meals.
- Think about meat substitutes like tempeh or tofu.

Moderation of Sodium:

Relevance: Consuming too much salt raises blood pressure, which increases the risk of coronary heart disease (CAD).

Management Tip: Steer clear of processed meals since they often contain excessive salt. Spices, herbs, and other flavorings may be used to improve the flavor of your food without using too much salt.

Rich in Antioxidants Foods:

Significance: Heart health is promoted by antioxidants, which are present in vibrant fruits and vegetables and fight inflammation and oxidative stress.

Management Tip: Arrange bright vegetables on a dish to make it stand out. Citrus fruits, leafy greens, and berries make great snacks.

Drinking plenty of water

Importance: Adequate hydration promotes general health and maintains ideal blood viscosity.

Management Approach: Drink eight glasses of water daily or more. Restrict your consumption of sugar-filled drinks and too much coffee.

Knowing how diet plays a part in treating CAD is about empowerment rather than limitation. It's about adopting a comprehensive and wholesome range of foods that build a lasting and pleasurable eating habit and strengthen the body. Making wise food choices allows you to contribute to the heart's health symphony actively, producing a tune of tenacity, grit, and long-lasting health.

Chapter: Fundamentals of Heart-Healthy Diet

2.1 A Heart-Healthy Diet's Significance

The Function of a Heart-Healthy Diet: Fueling the Core of Life

The heart is the hub of energy, the rhythmic force that directs the symphony of life in the vast tapestry of wellbeing. A heart-healthy diet becomes the conductor of this complex symphony, requiring each note to harmonize in a song of resilience and wellbeing. Together, we will explore the many benefits of a heart-healthy diet and how it serves as a deep form of self-care and a crucial life fuel source.

Developing Cardiovascular Hardiness:

Expressive Significance: A diet low in fat provides the cardiovascular system with the necessary nutrients to ensure normal functioning, acting as a loving embrace. It turns into a kind gesture recognizing the heart's ceaseless attempts to keep life alive.

Symbolism: Every satisfying mouthful echoes with the promise of sustenance, demonstrating the dedication to strengthening the heart against aging and modern living stresses.

Harmonizing the Macronutrient Melody:

Expressive Significance: The macronutrients—proteins, fats, and carbohydrates—have distinct functions in preserving a symphony of balance, much like notes in a musical composition. A heart-healthy diet aims to achieve a harmonic balance, where every nutrient plays a part without taking center stage.

Symbolism: Life in balance, when no element predominates, and all components cooperate to maintain the lovely rhythm of health, is symbolized by the balanced plate.

Reaping the Benefits of Plant-Based Music:

Expressive Significance: Plant-based foods such as fruits, vegetables, whole grains, and legumes are included as a lyrical ode to the planet's abundance. It represents a reconnection with nature, acknowledging the color and energy nutrients from plants provide the heart.

Symbolism: Every plant-based meal celebrates life's interdependence, a dance with the elements that nourish the body and spirit.

Protecting Against the Unhealthy Fats Discord:

Expressive Significance: Eating a diet rich in heart-healthy fats, such as those found in avocados, almonds, and olive oil, helps protect against the discordant notes of harmful fats. It is a pledge to keep items high in cholesterol at bay so as not to disturb the delicate balance of the arteries.

Symbolism: Selecting healthful fats becomes a parable about making deliberate decisions in life, where each option affects the whole composition of wellbeing.

Enjoying the Antioxidant Symphony:

Expression: Foods high in antioxidants are like the colorful soloists in the heart-healthy diet ensemble; they have a bright hue. They defend against oxidative stress, which may upset the delicate balance of the cardiovascular system.

Symbolism: Each experience in life is like a kaleidoscope of colors, flavors, and lessons added to the complex mosaic of wellbeing, and the same is true with antioxidants.

Every meal takes on a lyrical quality when consumed in the elegant language of a heart-healthy diet—as a gift to the heart and a song that speaks to the promise of vitality and the dedication to a life well-lived. It crosses over from the world of nourishment into the hallowed domain of self-care, where each mouthful aims to nourish the body and the core of a robust, healthy heart.

2.2 Crucial Elements for Heart-Healthy Nutrition

Crucial Elements for Cardiovascular Health: An Orchestra of Life

The pursuit of cardiovascular health is like an enthralling symphony in the grand scheme of human health, in which every vital nutrient plays a distinct and colorful note. Together, these nutritional virtuosos contribute to the beautiful beat of a prime heart. Join us on a melodic trip to discover them.

The Fatty Acids Omega-3:

Think of the soft swells on the ocean; it's the calming symphony that omega-3 fatty acids weave throughout the cardiovascular system. These vital lipids, plentiful in fatty fish like trout and salmon, dance elegantly to decrease cholesterol, lessen inflammation, and soothe the heart with heart-healthy effects.

Picture yourself enjoying a meal of grilled salmon, with every mouthful bringing the nourishing tune of omega-3s to life and creating a cardiovascular resilience symphony.

Fiber:

Picture a fully blooming garden to understand the essence of dietary fiber, which is a powerful force in the cardiovascular health symphony. Fiber is found in whole grains, fruits, and vegetables. It performs a virtuosic role in heart health by encouraging good digestion, decreasing cholesterol, and promoting beneficial effects.

Enjoy the crunch of a kale salad topped with berries and almonds, knowing that the fiber-rich combination will promote the healthy health of your heart.

Oxidants

To understand the essence of antioxidants, picture dawn throwing a warm light across the horizon. Antioxidants, which include vitamins C, E, and beta-carotene, are found in vibrant fruits and vegetables. They act as a barrier against oxidative stress, preventing cellular damage and preserving heart rhythm.

Enjoy a bowl of colorful mixed berries, where antioxidants dance in a brilliant ballet that gives every mouthful a shot of antioxidant power.

Potassium

To understand the significance of potassium in cardiovascular health, picture a river meandering through a verdant environment with ease. Potassium, which is found in abundance in sweet potatoes, spinach, and

bananas, conducts a flowing symphony that controls blood pressure and maintains the heart's regular beat.
Savor a potassium-packed smoothie made with bananas, spinach, and Greek yogurt. It's a delicious concoction that will keep your heart healthy at every turn.

The mineral magnesium

Magnesium plays a part in the cardiovascular symphony. Picture a peaceful, moonlight night. Magnesium, found in nuts, seeds, and leafy greens, helps maintain a gentle rhythm, control blood pressure, and support heart health in general.

Savor a trail mix high in magnesium with almonds, pumpkin seeds, and dark chocolate, creating a delicious mashup that will envelop your heart with its nourishing melody.

Vitamin K:

Picture a beautiful dance to understand the cardiovascular performance's vitamin K essence. Vitamin K, included in broccoli and leafy greens, is essential for blood clotting because it maintains a healthy balance between circulation and coagulation.

Take pleasure in a colorful quinoa and kale salad that is enhanced by the subtle nutritional beauty of vitamin K.
Let's appreciate the beautiful instances of these vital minerals in our culinary repertoire as we enjoy their symphony. Like notes in a song, every nutrient adds to

the overall theme of cardiovascular health, producing a lively, robust, and timeless symphony that resonates harmoniously through a heart's chambers.

2.3 Meal balance and portion control

Meal Balance and Portion Control: Mastering the Art of Culinary Harmony

Portion management and balanced meals are the expert conductors in the culinary symphony of health, crafting a harmonic composition that nourishes the body and fosters wellbeing. Together, we will explore the relevance of portion management and culinary creativity in creating meals harmonious with nutritional balancc. Let's go on a delectable trip.

The Portion Control Symphony:

Preciseness and Harmony: Consider portion management the subtle skill of leading a musical group. Finding the ideal balance between sating hunger and abstaining from excess is about accuracy. Portion management ensures that every component on the plate adds to the total nutritional score, much like a conductor leading all the other instruments.

Awareness and Mindfulness: Mindfulness takes the role of the conductor's baton. Pay attention to your body's signals, enjoy every mouthful, and recognize the differences between fullness and hunger. Controlling portion sizes is about enjoying a feast with awareness and respect for the body's natural cycles, not about doing without.

What Makes a Balanced Lunch:

Proteins as the Melodic Foundation: Consider proteins as the piece's main melody. Proteins from lean meats, poultry, fish, beans, or tofu provide the essential amino acids and build a strong foundation for general health. Proteins provide solidity to balanced meals, just as they do to a symphony.

Harmonizing with Vibrant Produce: Picture a flash of color acting as the vivid brass and strings in a piece of music. Rich in vitamins, minerals, and antioxidants, fruits and vegetables provide a rainbow of nutrients and tastes. A symphony of health benefits is inevitable when you fill your plate with diverse, colorful food.

See Grains and Carbs as Harmonious Rhythms: See grains and carbs as the composition's sustaining rhythms that provide rhythm. Choose whole grains for a consistent energy source, such as quinoa, brown rice, or oats. The secret is to choose complex carbs that support a steady, well-balanced beat.

Think of healthy fats in nuts, avocados, and olive oil as the flavorful crescendo that gives a symphony depth and richness. These fats enhance cardiovascular health and give meals a delightful richness. The secret is to use the crescendo sparingly so it complements the music rather than overpowers it.

Techniques in Cooking:

Sauteing and Searing: Consider the culinary methods of sautéing and searing as imparting a pleasant crispness and depth of taste akin to the exactitude of musical articulation. These techniques make it possible to prepare delectable meals with little additional fat.

Steaming and Roasting: See steaming and roasting as methods that protect the nutritional value of food in the same way as musical notes are carefully preserved. These techniques guarantee a nutrient-rich harmony on your plate by keeping the vibrant tastes and colors of the veggies.

The Technique of Plating:

Presentation as Expression: Consider the visual representation of a culinary masterwork as the art of plating. The thoughtful arrangement of hues, textures, and sections on the plate resembles how a musical score is composed.

A well-presented food is not only inviting to taste and appreciate the symphony of tastes, but it also looks good.

Using Your Innate Tastebuds

Listening to Your Body: Visualize intuitive eating as having the capacity to pay attention to the inherent rhythm of your body, akin to picking up on the minute details of a music composition. You may construct a customized culinary piece that suits your unique requirements and tastes by paying attention to indications of hunger and fullness.

Every plate becomes a canvas for culinary creativity regarding portion management and well-balanced meals—a symphony of tastes, textures, and nutrients that uplift the senses and feed the body. Adopting portion control and creating well-balanced meals helps create a positive connection with food and a harmonious symphony of well-being that flows with your life's beat.

Chapter 3 Building a Heart-Friendly Kitchen

3.1 Stocking Ingredients That Are Heart-Healthy

Keeping Heart-Healthy Foods on Hand: Creating the Vitality Pantry

The kitchen is transformed into a hallowed place on the culinary path toward heart health—an alchemy workshop where the transformation of elements creates colorful, nourishing meals. Choosing a suitable color scheme for a painting is similar to the artistic process of storing heart-healthy supplies. Let's take a tasteful journey together, appreciating the importance of every component as they blend to create the harmonious composition of life.

Bright Vegetables and Fruits:

The Essence of Color: As you fill your kitchen with various fruits and veggies, picture the kaleidoscope of a farmer's market. These jewels are not just ingredients; they are life itself, full of fiber, vitamins, and antioxidants. The more intense the color, the greater the nutritious value. Imagine a variety of bell peppers, crisp apples, and verdant greens—each a paintbrush representing a heart-healthy lifestyle.

Entire Grains and Antiquated Pleasures:

The Cornerstone of Sustenance: See whole grains as the cornerstone of your pantry, providing both cardiovascular health and energy sustainability. Ancient grains such as barley and farro, quinoa, brown rice, and oats provide a symphony of nutty tastes and textures. Imagine each grain as a note in the energetic tune as you seek these healthy grains.

Trim Proteins:

The Foundation of Power: Think of lean proteins as the sculptors of resilience and muscle. These foods—fish, lentils, skinless chicken, and plant-based proteins like tempeh and tofu—are the fundamental components that strengthen your body. Imagine the lentils cooking in the pot or the grill marks on a piece of salmon; each creates a work of art with power inside.

Heart-Healthy Fats:

The Beauty of Oils and Nuts: Think of heart-healthy fats as the lubricants that keep the circulatory system operating at peak efficiency. The richness of nuts and seeds, avocado oil, and olive oil are not simply ingredients; they are the elixirs that infuse your recipes with taste and depth. Imagine a sprinkle of golden olive oil and the crunch of almonds, a delicious addition to your arsenal of heart-healthy foods.

Spice Rack Orchestra:

The Ballet of Flavor: Consider your spice cabinet a symphony of tastes, a trove of fragrant herbs and spices that elevate everyday meals to unique culinary creations. Imagine the brilliance of citrus zest, cumin's earthiness, and cinnamon's warm embrace. These components are the conductors that bring the flavor of your heart-healthy meals to a new level.

Plant-Based and Dairy Alternatives:

The Creamy Cadence: Visualize your culinary composition's creamy cadence from plant-based or dairy substitutes. Almond milk, tofu, and Greek yogurt are just a few of the ingredients that provide a symphony of nutrients and a luxurious texture. To illustrate how versatile these alternatives are, picture the smooth mix of a plant-based smoothie or the creamy texture of a yogurt parfait.

Herbs and New Fragrances:

The Fragrance of Wellbeing: Picture the aromas of fresh herbs filling your kitchen and giving your food life. Not only decorations, basil, cilantro, mint, and thyme are the aromatic whispers of health. Envision the cutting board as a platform where these herbs perform, unleashing their fragrant enchantment into your heart-healthy dishes.

As you fill your kitchen with these heart-healthy components, see each thing as a dynamic force that is part of your path toward wellbeing rather than just a member. The kitchen has evolved from a place for mundane chores to a haven where you can care for your body and spirit. By combining all the ingredients in your pantry, you are doing more than just cooking; you are producing a harmonious blend of health that flows with the cycles of life.

3.2 Recipes for Heart-Healthy Cooking

Cooking Techniques for Cardiovascular Health: A Wellness Culinary Ballet

The selection of cooking techniques in the culinary dance of heart health is a choreography of tastes, textures, and nutrients. Every method is a dance that carefully transforms components into a vibrant symphony. Let's take a graceful tour of the kitchen, showcasing the ways that not only maintain the heart-healthy properties of the products but also bring them to the pinnacle of culinary brilliance.

Steaming:

Imagine delicate tendrils of steam rising from a bamboo steamer, holding colorful veggies like carrots and broccoli. Steaming preserves food's nutrients, colors, and textures, creating a lyrical ballet. Vegetables are embraced by the dance of steam, which leaves them colorful, crisp, and full of heart-healthy nutrients.

Grilling

Picture flames slowly licking the surface of a piece of lean chicken or vibrant bell peppers over a hot grill. Grilling is the fiery waltz that gives vegetables and meats a smokey appeal. The grill's embracing of heart-healthy options is mingled with the seductive beauty of searing heat that seals in tastes without overdosing on fat.

Cooking and Baking:

Imagine a golden-brown symphony—a tray of roasted sweet potatoes or a delicious salmon fillet—coming out of the oven. Baking and roasting are the slow waltzes of cooking, enveloping food in a dry heat that intensifies tastes and creates a perfect combination of textures. This culinary dance highlights lipids that are good for the heart while maintaining the nutritional value of each component.

Sautéing:

Imagine an olive oil and garlic skillet coming to life, turning a mix of veggies into a delicious treat. Sautéing is a vibrant cooking technique that involves quickly cooking food in a tiny quantity of heart-healthy oil. The pan becomes a stage where flavors emerge quickly, producing a colorful and nourishing show.

The act of poaching

Imagine a saucepan slowly cooking and holding a juicy pear or a tender piece of fish. Poaching is a delicate culinary technique that involves immersing components in a simmering liquid to produce a soft and heart-healthy dish. The liquid used for poaching turns into a fragrant infusion that improves the overall flavor profile without sacrificing nutritious content.

Stir-frying:

Imagine a wok full of vibrant veggies, lean protein, and a harmonious blend of ginger and soy sauce. Stir-frying is a vigorous cooking method in which ingredients are quickly tossed over high heat while maintaining their nutritional value and crispness. This cooking demonstration highlights the skill of rapid, heart-healthy cooking.

Uncooked Preparations:

Imagine a colorful salad with a rainbow of fruits, nuts, and veggies. Raw dishes are the free-form ballet, where the ingredients are still as fresh and nutrient-dense as possible. A basic dish's symphony of tastes and textures celebrates heart-healthy abundance.

The kitchen is the stage, and the utensils are the instruments in this culinary dance for heart health. Every cooking technique is a beautiful ballet that honors the nutritional value of the ingredients while converting them into a masterpiece of deliciousness that is good for your heart. As you spin through these methods, picture your kitchen as a ballroom where the health dances with every graceful move, culminating in a gourmet creation that feeds the body and uplifts the soul.

3.3 Examining Food Labels and Choosing Wisely

Understanding Food Labels and Making Wise Decisions: The Craft of Interpreting Cooking Secrets

Understanding food labels turns into a compass that points us toward well-informed and health-conscious decisions while navigating the maze-like aisles of supermarkets, where items entice us with promises of taste and sustenance. Uncovering the culinary mysteries concealed inside packaging is a type of art, expertise, and literacy we possess. Let's take a trip through the language of food labels to discover the subtleties involved in making decisions that align with our overall health.

List of Ingredients:

Consider the components list as the canvas of a culinary masterpiece or the "Canvas of Composition." Every element is a stroke that adds to the composition as a whole. It takes skill to read the list and figure out the taste palette and nutritional harmony it contains. Seek for identifiable, healthful components and steer clear of additions that have been artificially or excessively processed.

Panel of Nutrition Facts:

The Nutritional Score Sheet: Consider the panel with nutrition statistics as a scorecard for your chosen foods. Calories, macronutrients, and micronutrients are the leading players in this. Making sense of these data and using them to guide choices is the art. Find a composition where the nutrients match your desired level of health. To guarantee an accurate nutritional evaluation, pay attention to serving sizes.

Serving Dimensions:

Portions as Portraits: See serving sizes as portraits that encapsulate the quantity of a particular dish that makes up a single portion. The frame contextualizes the nutritional information. The skill of interpreting serving sizes promotes mindful eating, curbs overindulgence, and increases portion awareness.

Sugars Added:

The Sweet Melody: If additional sugars were musical notes, the harmony of nutrition may be upset by an overabundance of them. Understanding the added sugars area means pursuing moderation in sweetness to ensure the meals we choose to support our health without overpowering our nutritional symphony.

Information about Allergens:

Think of allergy information as cautionary markers along the culinary highway. By reading this section, you may avoid substances that might be harmful to your health. Ensuring our decisions align with our unique dietary requirements and health concerns is an art of awareness.

Value Percentage (%DV):

The Nutritional Compass: See the percentageDVD as the compass directing you toward a nutrient-balanced path. Assessing how a particular meal fits your daily nutritional demands is an art of proportion, which you may practice by reading this section. Please use it as a guide to steer toward meals that are good for your general health.

Promotional Statements:

Culinary Sirens: Imagine marketing slogans as captivating tunes that draw us into the realm of product attraction. Reading these promises skeptically takes skill and distinguishing between nutritional truth and marketing hype. Look for verified claims and steer clear of overly optimistic ones.

Making educated decisions and reading food labels includes self-care, knowledge, and empowerment. Once learned, it's a language that lets us understand the culinary narratives packaged products tell. Allow the skill of reading food labels to lead you through the aisles as you make decisions that will not only entice your palate but also provide your body and spirit with a harmonious balance of health.

Chapter 4: Scrumptious and Packed with Nutrient Recipes

4.1 Morning Eats to Kickstart the Day

Breakfast Recipes: A Symphony of Morning Vitality - Energize Your Day

Breakfast is a symphony that sets the tone for the rest of the day, not just a meal. Let's have a gastronomic adventure with meals that will tempt your taste senses and provide the fuel you need to face the day. This will fill your mornings with energy.

1. Breakfast Bowl with Quinoa:

Components:

- One cup of cooked quinoa
- half a cup of almond milk
- Strawberries, blueberries, and raspberries are mixed berries.
- A small handful of nuts (walnuts, almonds)

- A honey drizzle

Guidelines:

1. Almond milk and cooked quinoa should be combined in a dish.
2. Add your preferred amount of nuts and a handful of mixed berries.
3. For sweetness, drizzle some honey over the bowl.
4. Make sure that the flavors are distributed evenly by gently mixing the ingredients.
5. Savor the nuttiness of quinoa and the natural sweetness of berries and honey in this protein-rich morning dish.

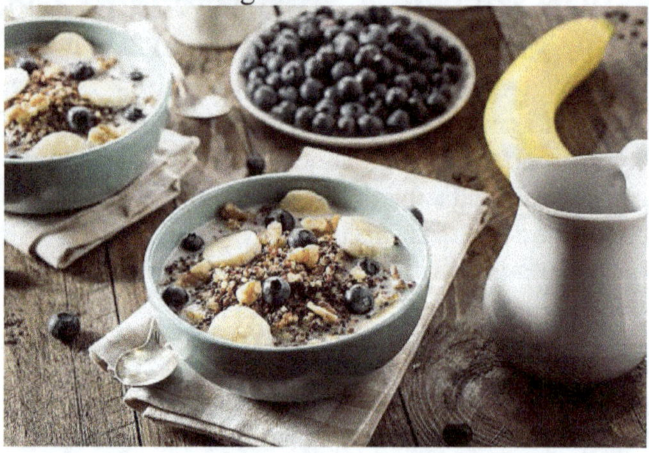

Harmony of Wellbeing: Picture a dish of cooked quinoa with a sprinkling of almonds and a colorful berry variety on top. Pour some honey over it to provide a hint of sweetness. This morning dish combines antioxidant-rich berries, crunchy almonds, and protein-rich quinoa for a well-rounded, energizing start.

2. Toast with avocado and a poached egg:

Components:

- Pieces of whole-grain bread
- ripe avocado
- a stolen egg
- Sliced cherry tomatoes
- To taste, add salt and pepper.

Guidelines:

1. Cuts of whole grain bread should be toasty to your taste.
2. Spread the mashed ripe avocado equally over the toast.
3. Place a flawlessly poached egg on top.
4. Add some cherry tomato slices as a garnish and season with salt and pepper.
5. Savor the perfect balance of fresh cherry tomatoes, a runny poached egg, and creamy avocado.

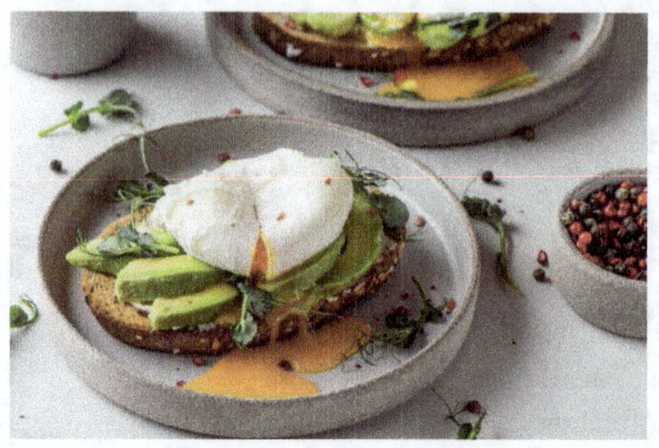

Morning Elegance: Picture a flawlessly cooked egg on top of whole grain toast, which has been spread with creamy avocado. Add cherry tomatoes, salt, and pepper as garnish. This breakfast is a work of art, combining protein, healthy fats, and a taste explosion that elevates the ordinary to the level of fine dining.

3. Greek Yogurt Concession:

Components:

- Greek yogurt
- granola
- Various berries
- Sweetheart

Guidelines:

1. Arrange Greek yogurt, granola, and mixed berries in a glass or dish.

2. Continue layering until you get to the top.
3. For sweetness, drizzle some honey over the parfait.
4. Savor the tastes and textures of this parfait, which combines crunchy granola, creamy yogurt, and a fresh burst of berries.

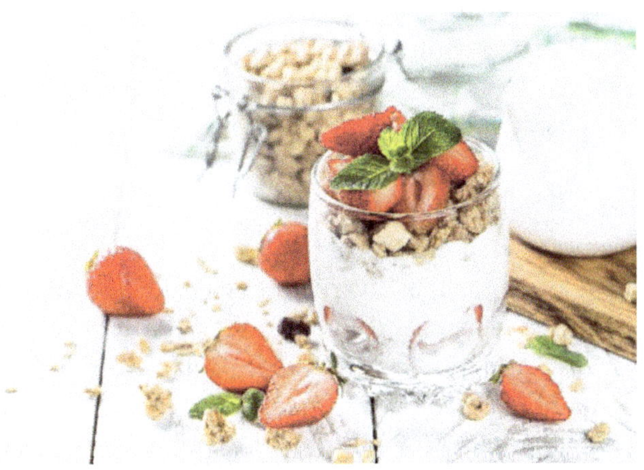

Layers of Vitality: Envision a glass filled with layers of luscious Greek yogurt, crisp granola, and a rainbow of berries. Add a honey drizzle for sweetness. This parfait is a symphony of textures, full of fiber, protein, and antioxidants. A pleasant trip through layers of morning vigor awaits you with every mouthful.

4. Feta and Spinach Omelet:

Components:

- Eggs
- fresh leaves of spinach
- Feta cheese, broken up
- Half a cherry tomato
- Olive oil
- To taste, add salt and pepper.

Guidelines:

1. In a bowl, whisk together eggs and add pepper and salt to taste.
2. Cherry tomatoes and fresh spinach should be sautéed in olive oil until they wilt.
3. Over the vegetables in the pan, pour the whisked eggs.
4. Top with feta crumbles and continue cooking until the omelet sets.
5. Serve the omelet, folding it over to reveal a delicious masterpiece of protein, veggies, and feta richness.

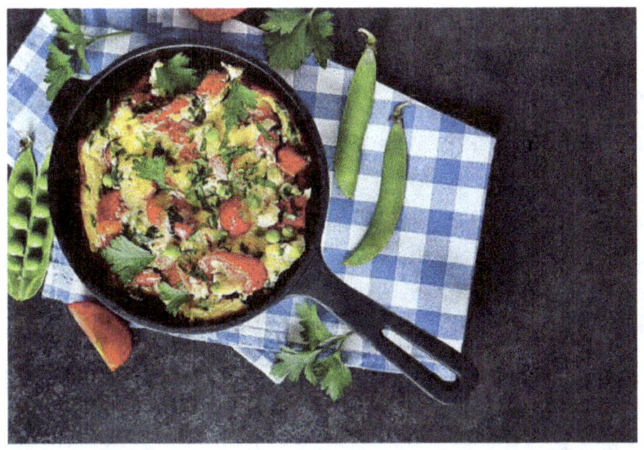

Omelette Sonata: Envision a fluffy omelette folded over a filling of sautéed spinach, crumbled feta, and cherry tomatoes. Cooked to perfection in a splash of olive oil, this omelette is a savory composition—a protein-packed masterpiece with the added benefits of leafy greens and the rich flavor of feta.

Smoothie Bowl:

Components:

- Berries that are frozen
- Banana
- a little handful of spinach
- Greek yogurt
- Almond milk
- Add-ons (granola, seeds, and nuts)

Guidelines:

1. Smoothly blend frozen berries, banana, almond milk, spinach, and Greek yogurt.
2. Transfer the blended drink to a bowl.
3. Add different textures to the top, such as granola, almonds, and seeds.
4. Savor the combination of the sweetness of fruits, the crunch of toppings, and the smoothness of yogurt in this nutrient-dense bowl.
5.

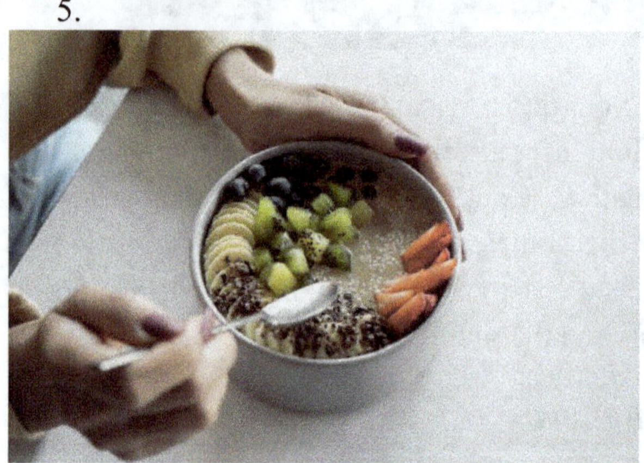

Smoothie Symphony: Visualize frozen berries, bananas, spinach, Greek yogurt, and almond milk all blending in a blender. Transfer into a bowl and garnish with granola, nuts, and seeds. This colorful smoothie bowl is a nutrient-dense concoction that combines yogurt's creamy creaminess, vitamins, and antioxidants.

6. Pudding with Chia Seeds:

Components:

- Chia seeds
- Almond milk
- extract from vanilla
- Maple syrup
- (Optional) Fresh Fruit

Guidelines:

1. Combine chia seeds, almond milk, maple syrup, and vanilla essence in a container.
2. Please give it a good stir, then chill for the night.
3. If desired, garnish with fresh fruit just before serving.
4. Savor the delicious pudding-like texture of chia seeds, which contain fiber, omega-3 fatty acids, and a little natural sweetness.

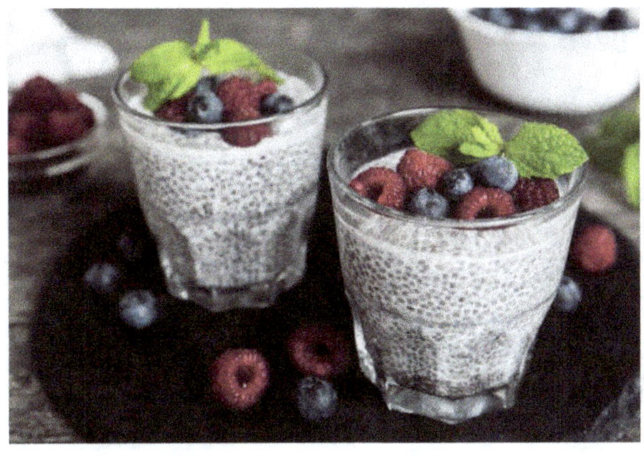

Chia Melody: Envision a jar full of soaked chia seeds in almond milk with maple syrup and vanilla extract sweetened. Add some fresh fruit on top. Packed with fiber, natural sweetness, and omega-3 fatty acids, this chia seed pudding has the texture of a lullaby. The exquisite combination of flavor and nourishment in every mouthful.

Berries with Whole Grain Pancakes:

Components:

- whole-grain flour
- Almond milk
- Eggs
- powdered baking
- Various berries
- Maple syrup

Guidelines:

1. Combine almond milk, eggs, baking powder, and whole-grain flour in a bowl.
2. To prepare pancakes, spoon some of the batter onto a heated griddle.
3. Place a heaping portion of mixed berries on top of the pancakes.
4. Pour some maple syrup over it for a bit of sweetness.
5. Savor the richness of maple syrup, the juicy berries, and the heartiness of nutritious grains.

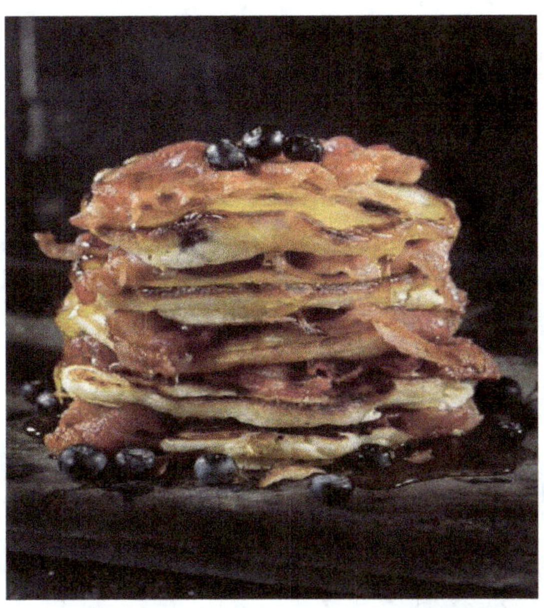

Pancake Sonata: Picture a pile of whole-grain pancakes with maple syrup drizzled on top and a waterfall of fresh berries. These pancakes are a morning staple, providing vitamins, fiber, and a hint of decadence. The robust grains provide you with steady energy for a vibrant morning.

A symphony of tastes, textures, and minerals, each of these breakfast dishes is meant to revitalize your day. Let the kitchen become your stage as you indulge in these morning treats; each word is a note in the health music that plays throughout your day.

Lunches for Long-Term Energy: An Afternoon Culinary Sonata

Lunch is a symphony that keeps us going until the afternoon's crescendo, not just a midday snack. A balanced combination of tastes and nutrients is necessary to achieve prolonged energy; it's like a culinary sonata that strengthens the body and the intellect. Together, we will explore various tasty lunch options that will satisfy our palates and offer us the long-lasting energy we need to get through the day.

1. Grilled chicken with quinoa salad:

Components:

- One cup of cooked quinoa
- Sliced, grilled chicken breast
- Vegetable mixture (cucumber, cherry tomatoes, and bell peppers)
- Feta cheese, broken up
- Olive oil
- Juice from lemons

Guidelines:

1. Combine cooked quinoa, grilled chicken pieces, and various vibrant mixed veggies in a sizable dish.
2. For an extra taste boost, top with crumbled feta.
3. To bring out the freshness, squeeze some lemon juice and drizzle with olive oil.
4. Gently toss the ingredients until well-mixed.
5. Savor the right blend of proteins, healthy grains, and colorful veggies in this nutrient-dense salad.

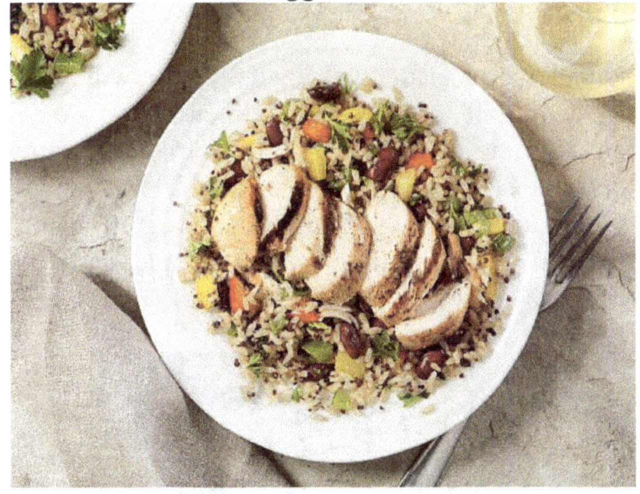

Balance of Proteins and Grains: Imagine a colorful quinoa salad with grilled chicken, mixed veggies, and feta crumbles on top. Add a dash of lemon juice and olive oil for a refreshing twist. This meal is a satisfying and energizing symphony of nutritious grains, crisp fresh veggies, and balanced meats.

2. Avocado and Salmon Wrap:

Components:

- whole-grain wrap
- Salmon fillet grilled
- Sliced avocado
- greens with leaves (arugula, spinach)
- Greek yogurt sauce

Guidelines:

1. On a level surface, place a whole-grain wrapper.
2. In the middle, put a cooked salmon fillet.
3. Add a handful of lush greens and some creamy avocado slices.
4. For a tart twist, drizzle with Greek yogurt sauce.
5. Tightly roll the wrap, cut it in half, and enjoy the health benefits of fiber, lean protein, and omega-3 fatty acids.

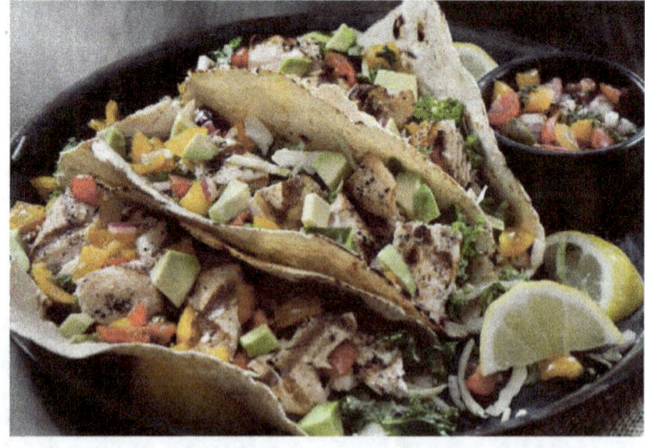

Oceanic Elegance: Picture a whole grain wrap stuffed with verdant greens, creamy avocado, and grilled salmon. Pour over some Greek yogurt sauce to add some taste. Rich in fiber, omega-3 fatty acids, and the healthful richness of whole grains, this wrap is a lunchtime ballet.

3. Buddha Bowl for vegetarians:

Components:

- cooked brown rice
- Rinsed and canned chickpeas
- Roasted veggies, such as carrots, broccoli, and sweet potatoes
- Sliced avocado
- dressing with tahini

Guidelines:

1. Place cooked brown rice in a bowl as the bottom layer.
2. Add avocado slices, roasted veggies, and chickpeas on top.
3. Drizzle with a large dollop of tahini dressing for a rich, delicious touch.
4. Gently toss to mix in all the ingredients.

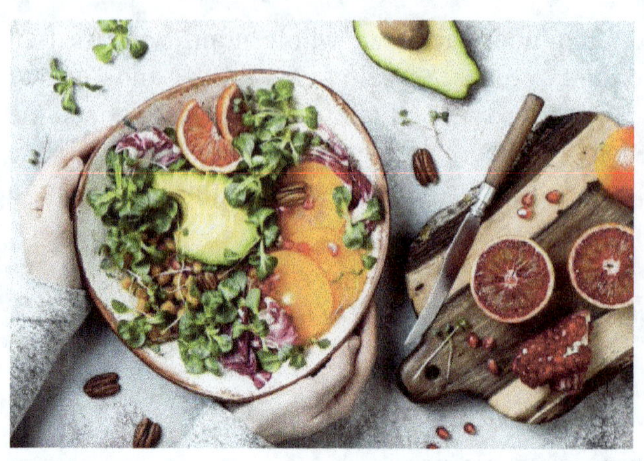

This plant-powered pleasure, a Buddha Bowl, offers a blend of healthful fats, plant-based protein, and fiber.
Imagine a dish full of roasted veggies, brown rice, chickpeas, and creamy avocado slices. This is a meal of nutritional harmony. Garnish with a luxurious tahini sauce. This Buddha bowl is a satisfying and energizing meal made of plant-based proteins, fiber, and the nutrients of vibrant veggies.

4. Stuffed bell peppers with turkey and quinoa:

Components:

- Cut bell peppers in half
- Turkey on the ground
- Cooked quinoa
- Caned and washed black beans
- Salsa
- Cheese in shredded form

Guidelines:

1. After preheating the oven, remove the bell peppers and place them in a baking tray.
2. Cook the ground turkey in a pan until browned.
3. Combine the turkey with the black beans, salsa, and cooked quinoa.
4. Place the combination of turkey and quinoa into the bell peppers.
5. Once the peppers are soft, sprinkle some shredded cheese and bake.
6. Savor the combination of lean protein, nutritious grains, and spicy salsa in these stuffed peppers.

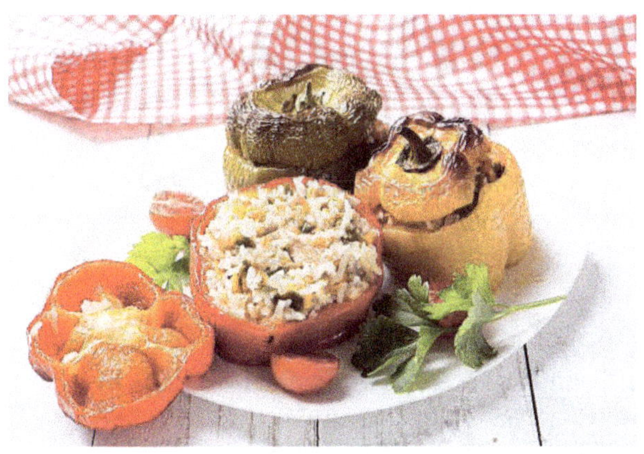

Imagine bell peppers filled with a blend of black beans, salsa, quinoa, and minced turkey, then covered with melted cheese to create a "stuffed pepper serenade." This meal is a culinary serenade, a satisfying and sustaining tune made with lean meats, nutritious grains, and salsa zing.

5. *Mediterranean Salad with Chickpeas:*

Components:

- Rinsed and canned chickpeas
- Half a cherry tomato
- Diced cucumber
- Feta cheese, broken up
- Sliced black or Kalamata olives
- Olive oil
- Juice from lemons

Guidelines:

1. Chickpeas, cherry tomatoes, chopped cucumber, crumbled feta, and sliced olives should all be combined in a dish.
2. For a Mediterranean taste profile, squeeze fresh lemon juice and drizzle with olive oil.
3. Gently toss the contents to ensure uniform coating.
4. The bright colors of the Mediterranean, together with plant-based proteins and healthy fats, combine to create a delightful salad.

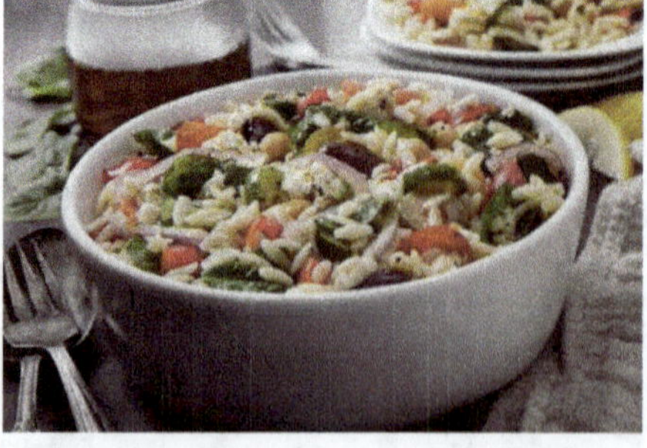

Imagine a colorful chickpea salad topped with cucumber, olives, crumbled feta, cherry tomatoes, and other Mediterranean flavors. Add a lemon squeeze and a drizzle of olive oil. This salad mixes plant-based proteins, healthy fats, and the vibrant freshness of Mediterranean tastes that awaken the senses. It is a Mediterranean song.

6. Stir-fried vegetables with quinoa:

Components:

- Cooked quinoa
- Various veggies, including snap peas, bell peppers, and broccoli
- Cubed tofu
- Soy sauce
- oil from sesame
- chopped ginger
- minced garlic

Guidelines:

1. Cubed tofu should be stir-fried till golden brown in a wok or pan.
2. To the tofu, add minced garlic, ginger, and mixed veggies.
3. Drizzle the mixture with sesame oil and soy sauce.
4. Stir in cooked quinoa and toss to mix well.

5. A satisfying dish of healthy grains, various veggies, and plant-based proteins, this stir-fry is a flavorful pleasure.

Stir-Fry Rhapsody: Picture quinoa, mixed veggies, and tofu in a vibrant stir-fry stirred in a flavorful concoction of sesame oil, soy sauce, ginger, and garlic. This stir-fry is a lunchtime symphony of a harmonious blend of plant-based proteins, fiber, and the fragrant undertones of Asian-inspired ingredients.

7. Salad de carne capers:

Components:

- Sliced, grilled chicken breast
- Half a cherry tomato
- Sliced fresh mozzarella
- fresh leaves of basil
- Balsamic reduction

Guidelines:

1. Place cherry tomatoes, fresh mozzarella, grilled chicken slices, and basil leaves on a platter.
2. Finish with a sweet and tart balsamic glaze drizzled over.
3. This salad, which has lean protein, mozzarella richness, and basil's fragrant freshness, is a masterpiece inspired by caprese.

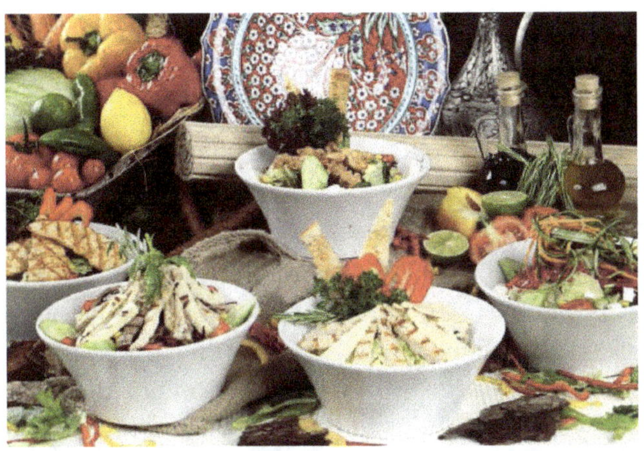

Caprese Crescendo: Picture a salad with balsamic-glazed grilled chicken, cherry tomatoes, fresh mozzarella, and basil leaves. A symphony of flavors, lunch is elevated with this salad, which is a Caprese crescendo composed of lean proteins, mozzarella richness, and basil's fragrant freshness.

These lunch dishes are more than simply meals; they're creations meant to satisfy hunger, increase energy levels, and boost productivity. Let the kitchen be your stage and these dishes your notes as you relish every mouthful; they're a symphony of tastes, textures, and nutrients that combine to provide sustained energy and vigor for the remainder of the day.

4.3 Tasty Dinners to Promote Heart Health

Dinner is a chance to create a symphony of tastes that connect with heart health, not merely the end of the day. Preparing meals focusing on cardiovascular health requires a thoughtful approach to cooking, a creative blend of nutrient-dense foods, and a healthy dose of flavor. Join us as we go on a gourmet trip via feasts that will excite your taste buds and nurture your heart with a gastronomic overture to wellbeing.

1. Salmon on the grill with a lemon-dill sauce:

Components:

- Filets of salmon
- Lemon
- new dill
- Olive oil
- minced garlic

Guidelines:

1. Set the grill's temperature to medium-high.
2. Salmon fillets should be seasoned with salt, pepper, and olive oil.
3. The salmon should flake easily with a fork after grilling it for 4–5 minutes on each side.

4. Combine the lemon juice, minced garlic, and freshly chopped dill in a small bowl.
5. Before serving, drizzle the grilled salmon with the lemon-dill sauce.

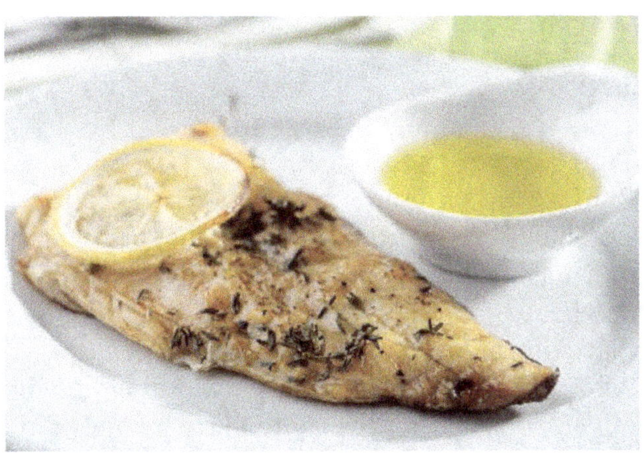

Marine Melody: Picture perfectly cooked, juicy salmon fillets with zesty lemon-dill sauce. This meal is a sea song made up of the freshness of the lemon, the perfume of the dill, and the omega-3 fatty acids from the salmon. It's a tasty tribute to heart health, not simply a meal.
With its crisp lemon and dill tastes and omega-3 fatty acids from salmon, this meal is a maritime symphony.

2. Bell peppers stuffed with Mediterranean flavor:

Components:
- bell peppers
- Cooked quinoa

- Rinsed and canned chickpeas
- chopped cherry tomatoes
- Feta cheese, broken up
- Olive oil
- Oregano

Guidelines:

1. Turn the oven on to 375°F, or 190°C.
2. Remove the seeds after halving the bell peppers.
3. Combine the cooked quinoa, chopped cherry tomatoes, chickpeas, and crumbled feta in a bowl.
4. Place the quinoa mixture into the bell peppers.
5. After sprinkling oregano and drizzling it with olive oil, bake it for twenty to thirty minutes.

To create a Mediterranean tapestry, imagine stuffing bell peppers with quinoa, chickpeas, cherry tomatoes, and crumbled feta. For a touch of the Mediterranean, drizzle with olive oil and sprinkle with oregano. This meal is a gastronomic masterpiece, combining fiber, plant-based proteins, and the depth of Mediterranean tastes.

This meal weaves fiber, plant-based proteins, and the depth of Mediterranean tastes to create a Mediterranean tapestry.

3. Herb-infused baked chicken breast:

Components:

- Breasts of chicken

- Rosemary
- thyme
- minced garlic
- Olive oil
- Zest of lemons

Guidelines:

1. Set oven temperature to 400°F or 200°C.
2. Add minced garlic, lemon zest, chopped rosemary, and thyme to chicken breasts for seasoning.
3. Pour olive oil over it, then bake for 20 to 25 minutes or until cooked.

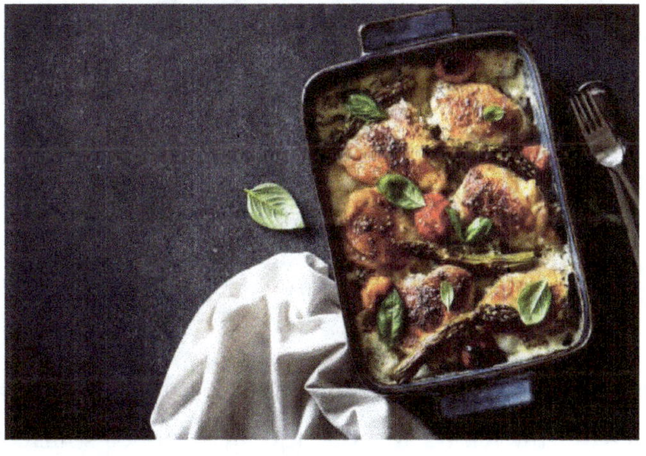

Herbaceous Harmony: Picture skinless, boneless chicken breasts roasted perfectly and flavored with garlic, thyme, and rosemary. Sprinkle some lemon zest on top and drizzle with olive oil. This meal is a showcase for lean protein with a pop of flavor that is both heart-healthy and fresh—a herbaceous symphony.

This herbaceous harmony is a heart-healthy, fresh taste explosion that showcases lean protein.

4. Plant-Based Lentil Soup:

Components:

- lentils
- Diced carrots
- chopped celery
- chopped onion
- minced garlic
- Broth made with vegetables
- chopped spinach

Guidelines:

1. Add the minced garlic and chopped onions to a saucepan and cook until fragrant.
2. Cook the chopped carrots and celery until they become tender.
3. Add the lentils and vegetable broth, then increase the heat until it boils.
4. After the lentils are soft, add the chopped spinach and simmer again.

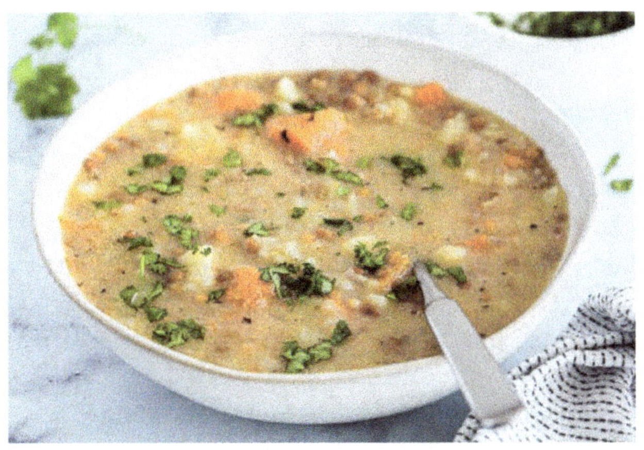

Soul-Warming Sonata: Picture lentils cooking in vegetable broth with carrots, celery, onion, and garlic in a pot. For freshness, add a handful of spinach. This meal is a comforting sonata for the heart and soul, made of fiber, plant-based protein, and a colorful blend of veggies.

This heartfelt sonata is a plant-based piece full of fiber, protein, and a rainbow of veggies.

5. *Primavera Whole Wheat Pasta:*

Components:

- Pasta made with whole wheat
- florets of broccoli
- Half a cherry tomato
- Sliced bell peppers
- Olive oil

- chopped fresh basil

Guidelines:

1. Follow the directions on the box to cook the whole wheat pasta.
2. Add the bell peppers, broccoli, and cherry tomatoes to a skillet and sauté them in olive oil.
3. Combine the cooked pasta and the steamed veggies.
4. Throw some fresh basil on top.

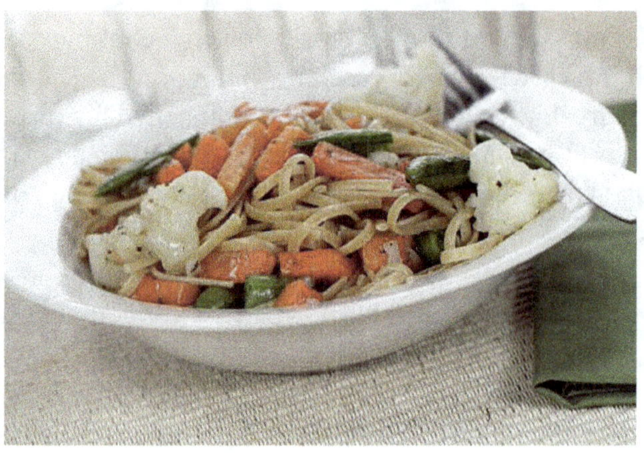

Imagine whole wheat spaghetti tangled with colorful bell peppers, cherry tomatoes, and broccoli. This is called pasta serenade. Add a drizzle of olive oil and sprinkle some fresh basil on top. Dinner tonight is a bright veggie medley, healthful grains, and heart-healthy olive oil—a pasta serenade.

This pasta serenade is a celebration of vibrant veggies, hearty grains, and heart-healthy olive oil.

6. *Quinoa bowl with stir-fried vegetables and tofu:*

Components:

- Cooked quinoa
- Cubed tofu
- mixed veggies, such as snap peas and bell peppers
- Soy sauce
- oil from sesame
- chopped ginger
- minced garlic

Guidelines:

1. Stir-fry cubed tofu in a wok until golden brown.
2. To the tofu, add minced garlic, ginger, and mixed veggies.
3. Drizzle the mixture with sesame oil and soy sauce.
4. Stir in cooked quinoa and toss to mix well.

Asian Fusion Overture: Picture a vibrant array of veggies paired with stir-fried tofu in a quinoa dish. Add garlic, ginger, sesame oil, and soy sauce. This meal is an intriguing combination of Asian tastes, healthy grains, and plant-based proteins. It's like an entrance to Asian fusion cuisine.

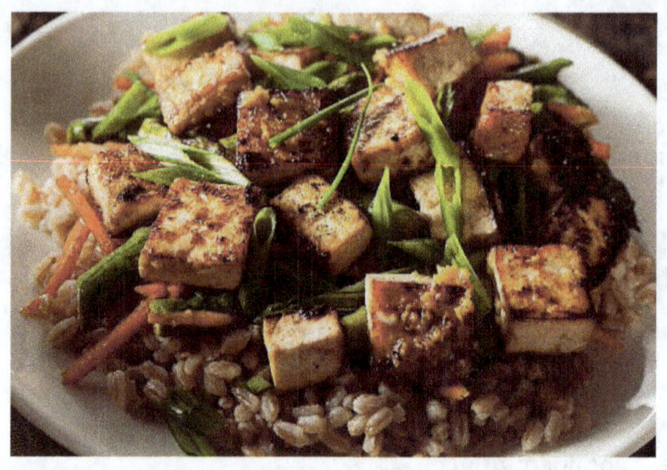

Combining nutritious grains, plant-based proteins, and the exotic appeal of Asian spices creates an Asian fusion entrée.

7. *Using tomato-basil salsa, bake the cod.*

Components:

- Fillets of cod
- Diced tomatoes
- chopped fresh basil
- finely sliced red onion
- vinegar with balsamic
- Olive oil

Guidelines:

1. Turn the oven on to 375°F, or 190°C.
2. After adding salt and pepper to the cod fillets, bake them until they are flaky and opaque.
3. Combine diced tomatoes, olive oil, balsamic vinegar, finely sliced red onion, and chopped fresh basil in a bowl.
4. Before serving, spoon the salsa made of tomatoes and basil over the baked fish.

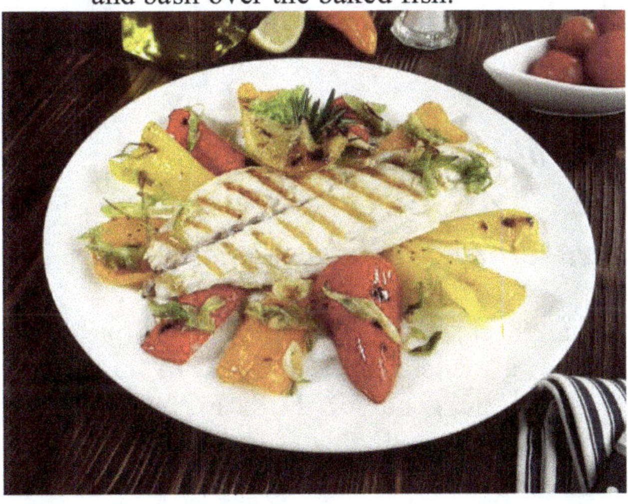

Asian Fusion Overture: Picture a vibrant array of veggies paired with stir-fried tofu in a quinoa dish. Add garlic, ginger, sesame oil, and soy sauce. This meal is an intriguing combination of Asian tastes, healthy grains, and plant-based proteins. It's like an entrance to Asian fusion cuisine.

With the fragrant freshness of basil and heart-healthy tomatoes, this salsa crescendo is a seafood pleasure.

Let the kitchen be your haven and each recipe a note in the symphony of wellbeing as you enjoy these heart-healthy feasts. These dinners are compositions meant to feed your heart and thrill your senses with a beautiful assortment of tastes, not simply food.

4.4 Sweet Treats & Snacks with a Heart-Healthy Spin

Heart-Healthy Twist on Snacks and Desserts: A Sweet Symphony for Cardiovascular Wellness

Desserts and snacks don't have to be guilty pleasures; they can be a delicious celebration of tastes and ingredients that are good for the heart. We'll look at snacks and desserts in this sweet symphony for cardiovascular wellness that satiates your desires and supports heart health. Let the kitchen become a scene where every morsel becomes a note in a conscious indulgence's music.

1. Dipped in Dark Chocolate Strawberries:

Components:

- Dark chocolate
- strawberry fresh

Guidelines:

1. Melt dark chocolate in the microwave or over boiling water in a heatproof basin.
2. Partially coat each strawberry by dipping it into the melted chocolate.
3. After dipping the strawberries, place them on a plate lined with parchment paper and cool until the chocolate sets.
4. Savor the natural sweetness of strawberries and the richness of dark chocolate.

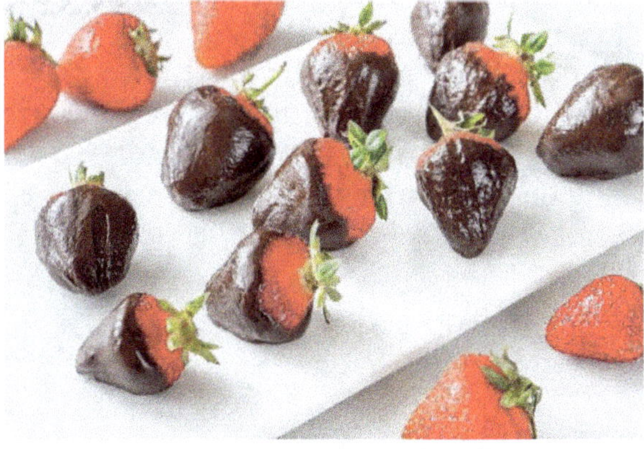

Think of juicy strawberries covered in luscious dark chocolate for an elegant take on chocolate. This dish is a masterpiece of chocolate elegance—a sugary confection that fulfills appetites and offers heart-healthy antioxidants from dark chocolate. Savor the elegance of this delicious dessert that is heart-healthy.

2. Trail Mix Nut and Seed:

Components:

- Walnuts with Almonds
- seeds of pumpkins
- Sunflower seeds
- Dried fruit (raisins, apricots)

Guidelines:

1. Combine almonds, walnuts, sunflower, and pumpkin seeds with your preferred dried fruit in a dish.
2. Mix the ingredients until well blended.
3. Divide the trail mix into portions that are the size of snacks.
4. Snacking on this nutrient-rich trail mix will keep your heart healthy.

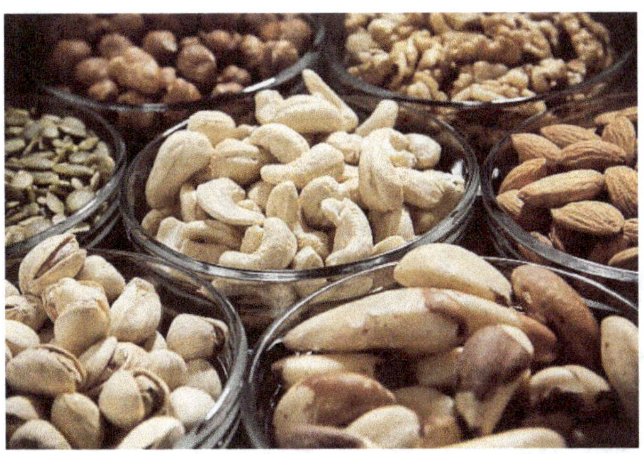

Imagine a combination of almonds, walnuts, sunflower seeds, pumpkin seeds, and dried fruits for the Trail Mix Sonata. This is a trail mix sonata, a combination of heart-healthy nuts and seeds that provide vital nutrients, including fiber and omega-3 fatty acids. Chew on this tasty blend for long-lasting energy and overall health.

3. Apple Chips with Baked Cinnamon:

Components:

- Apples Honey Cinnamon

Guidelines:
1. Turn the oven on to 200°F, or 93°C.
2. Using a mandoline or sharp knife, thinly slice the apples.
3. Place the apple slices on a baking sheet covered with parchment paper.
4. Drizzle with honey and sprinkle with cinnamon.

5. Bake until the apple slices are crispy, about 2 to 3 hours.
6. Enjoy the melody of the apple: it's crisp, delicious, and naturally sweet.

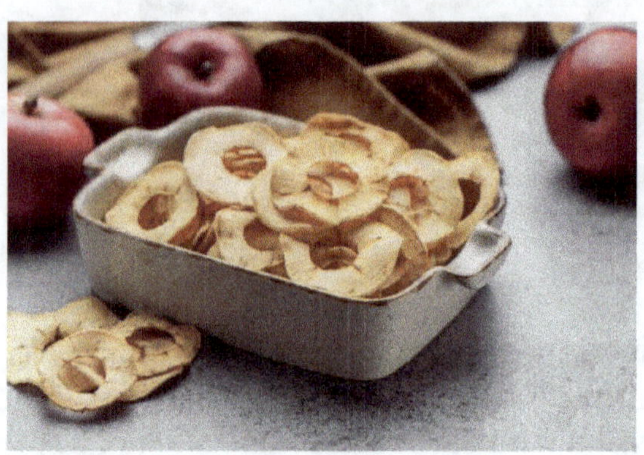

Apple Melody: Picture perfectly cooked, finely sliced apples sprinkled with cinnamon. This tasty and crunchy snack honors the inherent sweetness of apples with a delicious twist. It's an apple harmony. It's a heart-healthy substitute for candy since it has no added sugars.

5. Fresh Fruit with Chia Seed Pudding:

Components:

- Chia seeds
- Almond milk
- Extract from vanilla Maple syrup
- fresh fruit (mango, berries, etc.)

Guidelines:

1. Combine chia seeds, almond milk, maple syrup, and vanilla essence in a container.
2. Please give it a good stir, then chill for the night.
3. If desired, garnish with fresh fruit just before serving.
4. Savor the delicious pudding-like texture of chia seeds, which contain fiber, omega-3 fatty acids, and a little natural sweetness.

Imagine a jar full of soaked chia seeds in almond milk, sweetened with maple syrup and vanilla essence, and garnished with fresh fruit. This is the recipe for Chia Pudding Rhapsody. This dish is an improvisation of chia pudding, rich and nutrient-dense. This pudding is heart-healthy because chia seeds provide fiber and omega-3 fatty acids.

6. Chocolate Mousse with Avocado:

Components:

*   Avocado Powdered Cocoa
*   Maple syrup
*   extract from vanilla

Guidelines:

1. Smoothly blend ripe avocado, vanilla essence, maple syrup, and chocolate powder.

2. The chocolate mousse should be chilled for at least half an hour.
3. Enjoy the richness of avocado, a heart-healthy substitute for conventional mousse, and serve chilled.

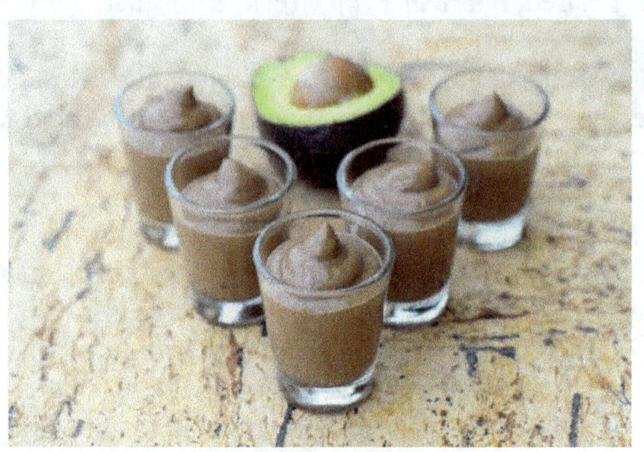

Mousse Crescendo: Picture a rich, velvety chocolate mousse composed of vanilla essence, maple syrup, cocoa powder, and ripe avocados. This dessert is mousse crescendo, a rich delicacy made with heart-healthy monounsaturated fats from avocados instead of saturated fats. Enjoy the wealth guilt-free.

7. Breakfast Cookies with Berries and Oatmeal:

Components:

- Oats rolled
- granary flour, Almond butter

- Blueberries and raspberries, or honeyberries

Guidelines:

1. Combine rolled oats, honey, almond butter, and whole wheat flour in a bowl.
2. Mix the cookie dough with the fresh berries.
3. Spoon dough onto a baking sheet in small sections.
4. Bake till golden brown along the edges.
5. Savor the coziness of these cookies, a harmonious combination of nutritious grains, nut butter, and the potent antioxidants in berries.

Cookie Symphony: Combine rolled oats, honey, almond butter, whole wheat flour, and berries in a bowl. The antioxidant power of berries, nut butter, and whole grains come together in a symphony of heart-healthy components in these cookies. Savor the comforting taste of cookies that improve cardiovascular health.

Let the kitchen become your haven as you make and savor these heart-healthy snacks and treats, where every dish is a note in the delicious symphony of mindful pleasure. Every mouthful of these meals celebrates flavor and health since they are designed with your heart's health in mind and taste.

Chapter 5: Modifying Your Lifestyle for a Heart-Healthy Heart

5.1 Including Exercise

Including Exercise: A Harmony of Motion for Optimal Health and Wellness

With our hectic schedules that often resemble a frantic crescendo, it is simple to lose sight of the significance of physical exercise in our everyday lives. However, in our hectic schedules, there is room for a transforming symphony—a well-balanced incorporation of movement that energizes the body and sets off a series of beneficial outcomes for our general wellbeing. Together, we will examine how to make physical exercise a part of your life, making every stride, pose, and breath sound beautiful.

The Wake-Up Dance as the Morning Prelude

Please think of the morning as your prelude to the day's symphony when the sun rises and casts its golden colors over the horizon.

Accept a slow dance of stretches, yoga positions, or a vigorous morning stroll. This wake-up dance awakens muscles, joints, and the mind simultaneously, balancing the body's systems.

Midday Interlude: Desk Work Duo

Discover opportunities to escape the monotonous routine of a sedentary existence amid the buzz of everyday duties and production.
Incorporate desk workouts into your workplace, such as shoulder rolls, sitting leg lifts, and stretches. This interlude brings your symphony of duties back to harmony while regaining circulation and reducing stress.

Sonata for Afternoon Allegro: Nature's Stroll

Nature beckons as the ideal background for a revitalizing walk in the afternoon when the day's energy is still total.
Take a leisurely walk around a local park, wildlife refuge, or neighborhood. As you walk quickly, let the sounds of rustling leaves and chirping create an allegro that uplifts your body and soul.

Mindful Movement Meditation in the Evening Adagio

Enjoy the peace of the evening as the day softly fades into darkness for a more reflective movement experience.
Take mindful movement exercises like tai chi, mild yoga, or a leisurely run. This adagio is a contemplative

lull before the night's curtain rises, encouraging calm and centering.

Dancing of the Stars, the Night's Finale

Let movement be your nightly celebration, a dance of energy under the stars, under the velvety shroud of darkness.
Pick pursuits that suit your interests, whether a moonlight jog, a dance party in your living room, or just some relaxing stretches before bed. This last section is a rhythmic release that lets the body know it's time to relax and let sleep heal.

Advice for a Harmonious Incorporation:

Make Movement Playlists: Make playlists that will help you feel more energized throughout the day and transform everyday tasks into a vibrant dance.

Include Loved Ones: Include family or friends to make physical exercise a shared experience. A group game or synchronized stroll adds a social element to your movement symphony.

Investigate Diverse Activities: To maintain the symphony of movement that is lively and captivating, vary your physical repertory by doing yoga, weight training, swimming, and cycling.

When incorporating physical exercise into your daily routine, think of it as a symphony rather than a chore—a collection of motions that improve your mood, nourish your body, and add to your overall wellbeing. Every stride, breath, and exercise contribute to the overall score of a vigorous, healthy life—a symphony that is entirely yours to lead.

5.2 Stress Reduction Methods

Stress Reduction Methods: Creating Calm in the Symphony of Life

Stress often takes center stage in life's chaotic symphony, so finding a balanced counterpoint is crucial. Stress management is more than just a coping strategy; it's an art form, a symphony of skills that, when carefully considered and performed with purpose, can turn the discord of stress into a calming tune of peace. Now, let's explore stress management approaches expressively, with each note helping to create a life that is resilient and peaceful.

Conscious Breathing: The Foundation of Being Present

The breath becomes the anchor in the middle of everyday pandemonium, a precursor that firmly establishes you in the here and now.

Breathe mindfully, taking deep breaths and letting them out gently. Breathe in a pattern that releases tension, enabling you to center yourself and clearly accept the present as it is.

Melodic Unwind: Progressive Muscle Relaxation

A discordant tone is created inside the body by tension that often becomes lodged in the muscles.

From your toes to your head, gradually tighten and then relax each muscle group. This soothing melody eases tension and creates a sensation of alleviate by encouraging bodily relaxation.

Imaginative Crescendo: Visualization

The mind longs for a visual diversion from the commotion, a crescendo of the imagination that whisks you away to a calm mental place.

Shut your eyes and picture a quiet location, such as a sunny beach, a calm woodland, or a serene mountain top. Give yourself up to the minutiae and let the creative climax to relieve tension.

Warm-Up: The Vibrant Prelude

Stress is often exacerbated by a sedentary lifestyle. The overture is movement, an exuberant lead-in to release tension.

Do something active on a regular basis, like dance, yoga, or running. Endorphins, the body's natural stress relievers, are released by the rhythmic movement, producing an energizing and upbeat symphony.

Journaling as a Form of Creative Expression

Stress may be increased by suppressing emotions. Writing in a journal becomes an artistic outlet—a vehicle for the song of the soul.

Keep a notebook where you may record your emotions, ideas, and reflections. This creative activity gives you perspective, assisting you in navigating your feelings and coming to peaceful conclusions.

Time Management: The Balanced Tempo

An uneven pace of life is often the root cause of overwhelm. Time management turns into the pace, a steady rhythm that guarantees every work has a place in the larger scheme of things.

Set reasonable objectives, prioritize your work, and divide more difficult activities into smaller, more doable jobs. The gradual increase in stress that results from an overfull schedule is avoided with this balanced pace.

Interconnectivity: The Melodic Group

Stress may intensify in isolation. The interaction of social ties that promotes emotional support is what makes connectivity into the harmonic ensemble.

Make deep bonds with your loved ones, friends, and support networks. In times of stress, depending on people and sharing your experiences together form a harmonic ensemble that provides comfort.

Suggestions for Harmonizing Stress Reduction:

Make routines: Whether it's drinking herbal tea, listening to calming music, or doing a little mindfulness exercise, create daily routines that promote calm.

Establish Limits: Acquire the ability to refuse when required. By establishing limits, you can save your time and energy and avoid a stressful spiral that gets out of control.

Accept Nature: Go outside and enjoy the melody of nature. The tranquil surroundings of nature provide a calming atmosphere for relieving stress.

Stress management strategies are the compositions that turn dissonance into harmony in the symphony of life. Every method is a note in the complex harmony of well-being, composing a calm tune that permeates your everyday life. When you incorporate these practices into your life, think of them not just as a way to deal with stress but as an ongoing orchestration—a never-ending symphony that leads you to resilience and calm.

5.3 Sustaining an Appropriate Weight

Keeping a Healthy Weight: The Craft of Living in Balance

Keeping a healthy weight requires more than simply the numbers on the scale; it requires a balanced lifestyle, attentive eating, and nurturing behaviors. We'll examine the nuances of keeping a healthy weight in this investigation of the art of balanced living, where each note stands for a deliberate choice that promotes general well-being.

Nutrient-Rich Composition: The Basis for Equilibrium

A symphony of health is created when the body is properly nourished.

Make a balanced diet high in whole grains, fruits, veggies, lean meats, and healthy fats your first priority. These nutrient-dense foods provide vital vitamins, minerals, and energy without adding extra calories, making them the cornerstone of maintaining a healthy weight.

Portion Control: Moderation's Harmony

Serving sizes have an impact on the total balance of calories consumed.

Take a careful approach to eating by observing portion proportions. Use smaller plates, chew your food thoroughly, and pay attention to your body's signals of hunger and fullness. The harmonic moderation of portion management guarantees a balanced daily intake of calories.

Water Symphony: The Wellbeing Elixir

The unsung hero of the body's everyday composition, hydration is essential.

The key to health is water. Drink enough water throughout the day since sometimes the body confuses dehydration for hunger. This hydration symphony promotes weight management and metabolic processes.

Consistent Exercise: The Vitality Dance

Engaging in physical exercise is vitality's dance and a crucial part of maintaining a healthy weight.

Exercise on a regular basis, including strength training with cardiovascular exercises (such as jogging, cycling, or walking). This energetic dance promotes general health, including cardiovascular and muscular tone, in addition to burning calories.

The Ingredients of Good Sleep: The Healing Serenade

Like a soothing lullaby to the body, getting enough sleep is essential for managing weight.

Aim for seven to nine hours of good sleep every night. Sleep affects appetite and satiety-related hormones, which in turn affects the way you choose to eat and manage your energy levels. A peaceful night's sleep is essential to the balance of maintaining a healthy weight.

Intentional Dining: The Meditative Art of Cooking

The gastronomic equivalent of meditation, mindful eating cultivates a strong connection between the mind and the senses.

Taste every meal and take note of its tastes, textures, and experiences. Recognize when your body is hungry and full, and while eating, stay away from distractions like devices. This mindful eating method promotes a healthy connection with food and increases awareness.

Emotional Wellbeing Group: The Encouragement Chorus

A vital component of the weight maintenance symphony is emotional well-being.

Create a nurturing emotional atmosphere. Weight control might be upset by emotional eating. Look for constructive ways to deal with stress, worry, or boredom, such spending time with friends, being attentive, or doing fun things.

Advice for Maintaining a Harmonious Weight:

Set Achievable but Realistic objectives: Make realistic objectives for maintaining your weight. Put more emphasis on your general state of well-being than you would on a particular scale number.

Celebrate Progress: Acknowledge and celebrate each little accomplishment you make. Honoring accomplishments encourages perseverance and fosters good conduct.

Remain Consistent: Reliability is essential for the weight maintenance symphony to flourish. Achieving long-lasting outcomes requires continuously establishing and maintaining healthy behaviors.

Keeping a healthy weight is like playing a multi-part composition in the symphony of health, where every note adds to the overall harmony. To build a symphony of well-being that echoes throughout your life, the art of balanced living entails embracing these notes: nutrient-rich choices, portion management, water, physical exercise, quality sleep, mindful eating, and emotional wellbeing.

5.4 Heart-Healthy Long-Term Routines

Long-Term Heart Wellness Routines: Creating a Cardiovascular Health Symphony

Forming enduring routines for heart health is like writing a classic symphony—one that reflects the values of exercise, nutrition, and awareness. Every habit you form along the path to a heart-healthy lifestyle becomes a note that blends together to create a song that promotes cardiovascular health. Let's examine the crucial enduring behaviors that support your heart's continued well-being.

Fulfilling Diet: The Perpetual Feast of Wellness

A diet rich in heart-healthy foods is a never-ending feast that sustains life.

Adopt a diet high in whole grains, fruits, vegetables, lean meats, and healthy fats. Restrict the amount of processed foods, added sugars, and salt. This never-ending feast of wellness gives your heart the vital nutrition it needs and lowers cholesterol.

Consistent Physical Harmony: The Circulation Dance

Engaging in physical exercise is like dancing in the circulation, since it maintains the heart's beat.

Exercise on a regular basis, combining strength training with aerobic exercises like running or walking. This movement symphony strengthens the heart, improves cardiovascular health, and fosters general energy.

Stress-Reduction Sonata: The Calm Melody

The discordant note that may impact heart health is chronic stress.

Use stress-reduction strategies including mindfulness, meditation, deep breathing, and doing enjoyable things. This musical method promotes serenity and lessens the damaging effects of stress on your heart.

A Reliable Sleep Serenade: The Restoration of the Night

Good sleep is the nocturnal rejuvenator, a heart-rejuvenating serenade.

Make getting 7-9 hours of good sleep every night a priority. Keep a regular sleep schedule, establish a relaxing evening ritual, and make sure your sleeping space is restful. This song promotes general wellbeing and cardiac health.

Harmony of Hydration: The Flow of Well-Being

Hydration is the fluidity of health, a steady stream that keeps everything in proportion.

Water should be consumed in moderation throughout the day. Staying hydrated promotes healthy circulation, lowers blood pressure, and keeps the heart working as the body's main pump as well as it can.

Cigarette-Free Crescendo: A Breath of New Life

The discordant crescendo that may alter the makeup of the cardiovascular system is smoking.

If you smoke, get help to stop. One of the most important things you can do for your heart health is to stop smoking. Living a tobacco-free life allows for better circulation and lowers the risk of heart disease.

Regular Check-Up Rhapsody: The Harmony of Prevention

The proactive care melody of preventative harmony is routine health check-ups.

Notes on Prevention: Make an appointment for routine checkups with your physician. Keep an eye on your cholesterol, blood pressure, and other cardiovascular risk factors. Preventive care is a rhapsody that guarantees early identification and treatment of prospective heart health problems.

Advice for Heart-Harmonic Wellness:

Develop Social Connections: Encourage deep relationships with loved ones. A significant note in the heart health symphony is social support.

Practice Mindful Eating: Include mindful eating techniques such as enjoying each mouthful and being aware of your body's signals of hunger and fullness.

Keep Yourself educated: Keep yourself educated about heart health, comprehend the elements that go into cardiovascular wellbeing, and make wise lifestyle choices.

Imagine your path of developing long-term heart-healthy habits as a symphony—a composition of decisions that align with the fundamentals of a heart-healthy lifestyle. All of your habits—healthy eating, regular exercise, managing stress, getting enough sleep, staying hydrated, giving up tobacco use, and getting regular checkups— play a part in the harmonious whole of your cardiovascular health. Continuously arranging these behaviors culminates in a masterwork—a long-lasting heart health symphony that enhances your life for years to come.